THE KETOGENIC DIET

THE ULTIMATE GUIDE FOR RAPID WEIGHT LOSS!

ANNETT HILL

copyright owner. Legal action will be pursued if this is breached.

<u>Disclaimer Notice:</u>

Please note the information contained within this document is for educational and entertainment purposes only. Every attempt has been made to provide accurate, up to date and reliable, complete information. No warranties of any kind are expressed or implied. Readers acknowledge that the author is not engaging in the rendering of legal, financial, medical or professional advice. By reading this document, the reader agrees that under no circumstances are we responsible for any losses, direct or indirect, which are incurred as a result of the use of information contained within this document, including, but not limited to, errors, omissions, or inaccuracies.

Table of Contents

Preface

If you've been struggling to lose your body fats and get that dream body; you need to stop whatever you are doing and read this. Because this book reveals the ONLY way to speed up your weight loss process safely and EFFECTIVELY.

In a couple of seconds, I'm going to tell you the 'accidental' diet discovered in 1924 designed to help children with epilepsy turns out to be a breakthrough for weight loss! You will discover how to turn your body into a 24/7 fat burning machine. Also, will help you reach your Fitness goals sooner than you could ever imagine!

****

WHY ARE YOU STILL STRUGGLING WITH WEIGHT LOSS?

****

If you have been struggling to lose weight even if you have been exercising regularly, this could be the ONLY solution for you.

Here is why:

No matter how frequently you exercise.

You will NOT lose weight if your body is NOT in a Fat-burning mode. Sadly, most people start exercising with the expectation to lose weight fast. Of course, exercising will help you to lose weight and be healthy, but it is NOT the fastest way to lose weight. However, if you combined exercise and follow the 'Right' diet, you will be able to lose weight FAST. This diet will 'trick' your body into a 24/7 burning machine by making it use your stored body fats as an energy source instead of using carbs in your bloodstream.

The good news is this is entirely safe and easy to follow and will shortcut your way for rapid weight-loss. Well, today is your most important day. I am going to reveal to you the diet that will help you to turn your body into a 24/7 fat burning machine so that you can even burn fat while you sleep!

There is no way in the world you will find a better strategy for rapid fat loss. This scientifically proven & tested weight loss diet is THE REAL DEAL.

Today, I am going to share with you the Ultimate Diet that helped me to shed away my stubborn body fats, feeling healthier and happier. Now is the time for you to do the same.

Your frustration ends here.

This might be the ONLY solution you have been looking for. Considering that, you will be able to:

- Turn Your Body Into A 24/7 Fat Burning Machine

- Be Healthier, Happier & Fitter

- Be At Your Very Best Self, Physically and Mentally.

- Have A High Mental Focus To Be Productive At Work

- Live Longer And Become A Cancer-Proof Superhuman

- Melt That Stubborn Belly Fat

- Most Important, You Will Reach Your Fitness Goals Much Sooner Than You Think!

Introducing.

Ketogenic Diet. The Complete Health & Rapid Fat Loss Diet Blueprint. Researches have been made that proves the Ketogenic Diet cannot only help with weight loss but to treat other diseases such as Epilepsy,

High Blood Pressure, Diabetes and even Cancer!

You get to reap all the health benefits of Ketogenic Diet as well as achieving your dream body. The time to transform your body is now!

Here is What You Will Learn From this Ketogenic Diet Blueprint:

- How Ketogenic Diet Does Enhances Fat Loss?

- How To Turn Your Body Into A Fat Burning Machine All Day Without Going Into Starvation Mode

- The Only Side Effects of Keto Diet? (Hint: It's A Good Side Effect)

- 8 'hidden' Benefits Of Keto Diet Other Than Losing Weight Easily

- How To Eliminate Sugar Spikes For Diabetic People Once And For All

- How To Get Higher Mental Focus

- How To Improve Your Memory

- Avoid The Types Of Food That Can Cause 'Foggy' Brain.

- How To Increase Energy Level Without Relying On 'Sugar Rush.'

- How to Get a Clearer, Healthier and More Glowing Skin in a Matter of Weeks.

- 4 Ways Ketogenic Diet Destroy Cancer Cells

- 8 Central Food To Eat And To Avoid On A Ketogenic Diet

- Why You Should Switch From Paleo To Keto Diet

- Will Keto Diet Affect Your Athletic Performance?

- 10 Easy Steps On Getting Started With Keto Diet

- 18 Yummy Keto Recipes That You Can Easily Prepare. And so much more waiting to be uncovered inside!

That is just scratching the surface!

Serious about transforming your body!

The good news is. You are just one step away from getting the body that you wanted.

All you have to do is to just apply this diet to start turning your body into a 24/7 fat burning machine for the next 30 days.

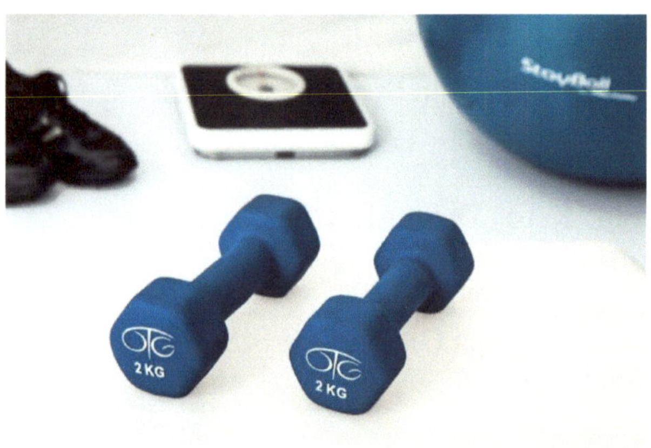

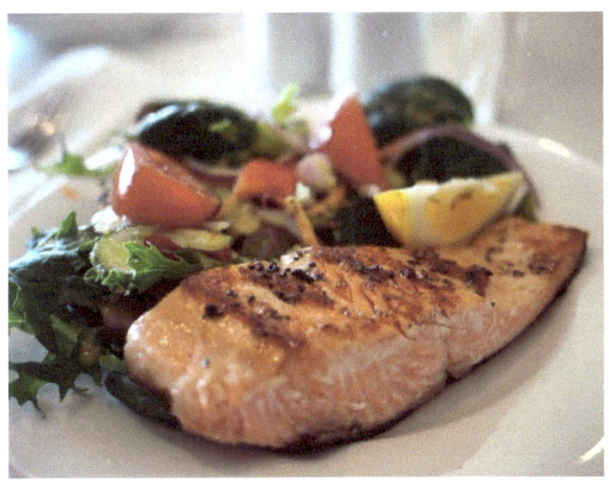

Introduction

Although the ketogenic diet has been around for almost a century, it is rapidly gaining popularity today. There is a reason why keto is so highly regarded. It is not a fad diet. It works, and it has tremendous health benefits in addition to weight loss. When on the keto diet, you are feeding your body precisely what it needs, while eliminating toxins that will slow it down.

The keto diet focuses on low carbohydrates, which the body converts into energy to help speed up weight loss. What exactly is the problem with high carbs, and why should you avoid them? Carbohydrates are converted into glucose and cause a spike in insulin. As the insulin enters the bloodstream to process the glucose, which becomes the primary source of energy. A spike in insulin can also result in storage of fats. The body uses carbohydrates and fats as energy, the former being the primary source. Therefore, the more carbs you consume in your daily diet, the less fat is being burned for energy. Instead, the spike in insulin will result in more fat storage.

When you consume fewer carbohydrates, the body goes into a state referred to as ketosis. Thus, the name for this low-carb diet. Ketosis helps the body survive on less food. By being in ketosis, you 'train' your body to utilize fats as the primary source of energy instead of carbs, just because there is close to zero carbs, to begin with. During ketosis, the liver breaks down fats into ketones; this enables the body to use the fat as energy. During a keto diet, we do not starve ourselves of calories; we starve the body of carbohydrates. This makes weight loss easy and natural. Later on, you will learn that the keto diet has many additional health benefits besides fat loss.

The keto diet is an easy diet, but some people do miss beans and bread. It takes a bit of getting used to, starting anything new is challenging after all. Ultimately, you will feel much better, both physically and mentally that you would be happy to avoid carbs finally. Also, being able to eat bacon on a diet does have its rewards!

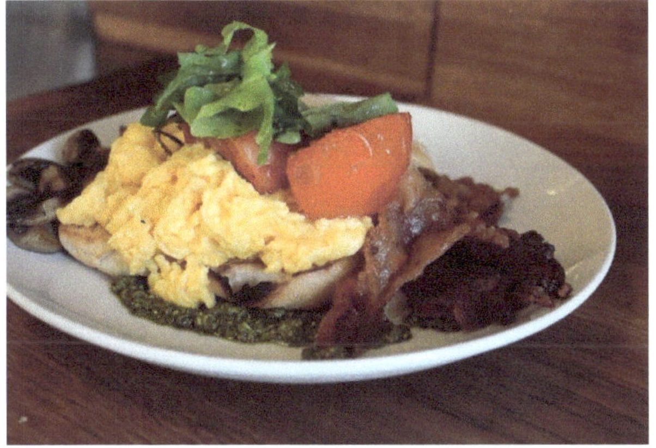

CHAPTER 1

WHAT IS
KETOGENIC DIET?

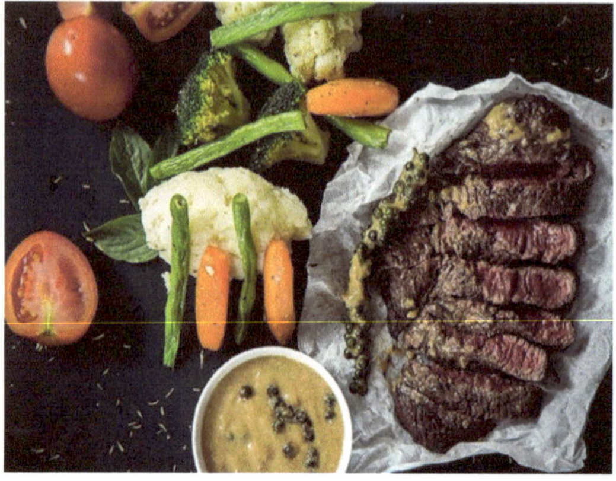

What is the Ketogenic Diet?

The keto diet is a low or zero carbohydrate diet, but it differs from other low-carb diets (such as Paleo) in that it deliberately manipulates the ratios of carbs, fats, and protein to switch fat into the body's primary source of fuel. Our bodies are used to using carbohydrates as fuel. Fats, which are a secondary source of fuel, are rarely tapped on. That means the extra fat is stored and keeps adding on the pounds.

The only ways to reduce fat in a 'normal' diet are to consume less fat and workout a lot to increase energy expenditure over daily calories intake, which is why most people fail to lose weight on the conventional diet.

On the other hand, the ketogenic diet uses fat for fuel, which means it gets used instead of being stored. So, weight loss becomes easy. In addition to weight loss, the ketogenic diet is known as the "healing" diet. The lack of sugar intake has been proven to help and prevent many diseases such as heart disease, high blood pressure, cancers, epilepsy, and many symptoms of aging.

The manipulation of carbs, fats, and protein is crucial to get into ketosis. It is a state when the body, deprived of the usual carbohydrates and sugar, is forced to use fat as its primary fuel. Therefore, the ratio of fats and protein are significantly higher than carbs in general.

Of course, consuming fewer carbs also means lowering the amount of insulin in your body. Also, Less insulin, less glucose and fat storage. That is why the keto diet has been so successful in helping people with diabetes. It adjusts the sugar level naturally.

The ratio of carbs, fat, and protein can vary. Many people allow themselves up to 50 grams of carbohydrates a day and still lose weight. On a stricter regime, the carb intake can be between 15 and 20 grams daily. The fewer carbs, the quicker the weight loss, but the diet is very flexible.

On the keto diet, you do not count calories. You count carbohydrates and adjust the intake of carbs vs. fat and protein. A typical keto diet will get 60 percent of its calories from fat, 15 to 25 percent of calories from protein, and 25 percent of calories from carbohydrates. The only limitation on the diet is sugar, which you need to avoid.

The ketogenic diet is not a fad. Many scientific studies have shown the benefits and healing effects of ketosis. Discuss the ketogenic diet with your doctor if you are interested in consuming less sugar, losing weight, or as preventive measures against vulnerable health problems.

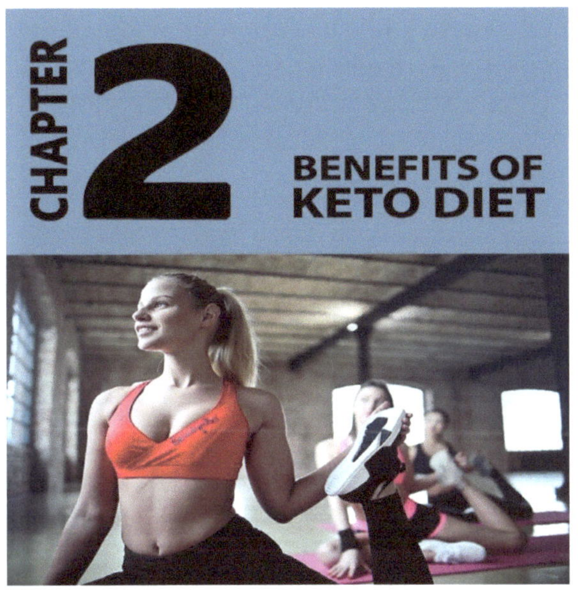

Benefits of the Keto Diet

Although ketogenic diet is popularly known as a 'rapid fat loss diet,' it is more to this than meets the eye. In fact, weight loss and higher levels of energy are only by-products of the keto diet, a kind of bonus. It has been scientifically proven that the keto diet has many additional medical benefits.

Let us begin by stating that a high carbohydrate diet, with its many processed ingredients and sugars, has no health benefits. These are merely empty calories, and most processed foods ultimately serve only to rob your body of the nutrients it needs to remain healthy. Here is a list of actual benefits for lowering your carbohydrates and eating fats that convert to energy:

Control of Blood Sugar

Keeping blood sugar at a low level is critical to manage and prevent diabetes. The keto diet has been proven extremely effective in preventing diabetes. Many people who have diabetes are also overweight. That makes an easy weight-loss regime a natural. However, the keto diet does more. Carbohydrates are converted to sugar, which for people with diabetes can result in a sugar spike. A diet low in carbohydrates prevents these spikes and allows more control over blood sugar levels.

Mental Focus

The keto diet is based on protein, fats, and low carbohydrates. As we have discussed, this forces fat to become the primary source of energy. This is not the typical western diet, which can be quite deficient in nutrients, particularly fatty acids, which are needed for proper brain function.

When people suffer from cognitive diseases, such as Alzheimer's, the brain is not using enough glucose, thus becomes lacking in energy, and the brain has difficulty functioning at a high level. The keto diet provides an additional energy source for the brain.

A study by the American Diabetes Association found that Type 1 diabetics improved their brain function after consuming coconut oil. That same study indicated that people who have Alzheimer's might experience enhanced memory capacity on a keto diet. Those with Alzheimer's have seen improved memory scores that might correlate with the amount of ketones levels present.

What does this study mean to an average person? With the emphasis on fatty acids, such as omega 3 and omega 6 found in seafood; the keto diet is likely to fuel the brain with the additional nutrients to help achieve a healthier mental state. The brain tissue is made up mainly of fatty acids (you have heard fish referred to as "brain food"), and the increased consumption of those fatty acids will logically lead to improved brain health.

Our body does not produce fatty acids on its own; we can only obtain it through our diet. Also, the keto diet is rich in fatty acids. A diet high in carbohydrates can lead to a "foggy" brain, where you have difficulty focusing. Focusing becomes easier with the increased energy provided by the keto diet. In fact, many people who have no need or desire to lose weight use the keto diet to improve and enhance brain functions.

Increased Energy

It is not unusual, and has become almost standard, to feel tired and drained at the end of the day because of a poor, carbohydrate-laden diet. Fat is a more efficient source of energy, leaving you feeling more vitalized than you would on a "sugar" rush.

Acne

While most of the benefits of a keto diet are well documented, one advantage catches some people by surprise: better skin and less acne. Acne is common. Ninety percent of teens suffer from it, and many adults do, as well.

While it was always thought that poor diet at least exacerbated acne, controlled research is still being conducted. However, many people on the keto diet have reported clearer skin. There may be a logical reason. A 1972 study found that high levels of insulin could cause the eruption of acne. Since a keto diet keeps insulin at a low and healthy level, it may very well affect skin health.

Besides, acne thrives on inflammation. The ketogenic diet eases and reduces inflammation, thus enabling the body to decrease acne eruptions. Fatty acids, which are found in abundance in fish, are a known anti-inflammatory.

While research is still being done, it seems likely that a keto diet has beneficial effects for brighter, healthier, more glowing skin.

Keto and Anti-Aging

Many diseases are a natural result of the aging process. While there have not been studies done on humans, studies on mice have shown brain cell improvement on a keto diet.

Several studies have shown a positive effect of the keto diet on patients with Alzheimer's disease. What we do know is that a diet filled with proper nutrients and antioxidants, low in sugar, high in protein and healthy fats, while low in carbohydrates, enhances our overall health. It protects us from the toxins of a poor diet.

There is also research indicating that using fatty acids for fuel instead of sugar may slow down the aging process, possibly because of the adverse effects that sugar has on our overall wellbeing. Also, the simple act of eating less and consuming fewer calories is a matter of basic health, as it prevents obesity and its inherent side effects.

So far, studies have been limited. However, considering the powerful positive effects of the ketogenic diet on our health, it is logical to assume this diet will help us grow older in a more natural way while delaying the natural effect of aging. A typical western diet laden with sugars and processed foods is undoubtedly detrimental to warding off the signs of aging.

Keto and Hunger

One of the reasons diets fail is hunger. People, who diet, feel hungry and deprived and give up. A low carbohydrate diet naturally leaves people feeling full and satisfied. Less hungry means, people will remain on the diet longer while consuming fewer calories.

Keto and Eyesight

People with diabetes are aware that high blood sugar can lead to a higher risk of developing cataracts. Since the keto diet controls sugar levels, it can help retain eyesight and help prevent cataracts. This has been proven in several studies involving diabetic patients.

Keto and Autism

We know the keto diet affects brain functions. In a study on autism, it concluded that it also has a positive effect on autism. Thirty autistic children were placed on the keto diet. All showed improved in autistic behavior, especially those on the milder autistic spectrum. While more studies are needed, the results were extremely positive.

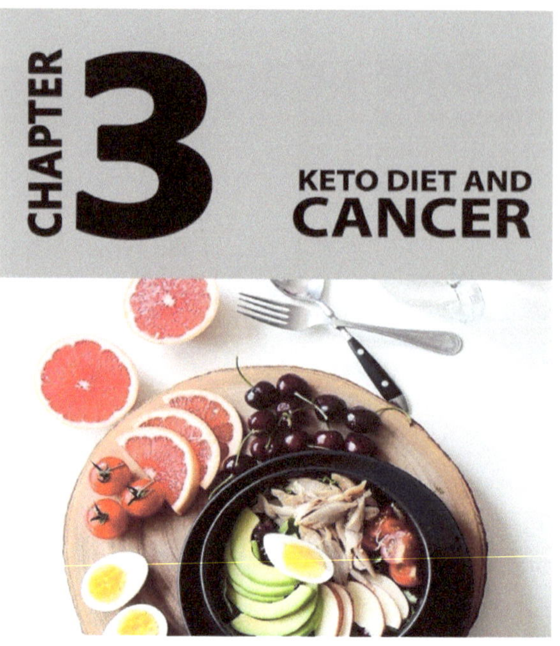

The Keto Diet and Cancer

Cancer has turned into a severe disease in our modern society. While cancer was not a significant factor before the 20th century (it did exist, of course), our modern diet and sedentary lifestyle have made cancer the second primary cause of death, with 1600 American dying from this disease every day. It appears that our bodies do not react well to being exposed to daily toxins.

While your physician must guide any cancer treatment, it is a good idea to discuss the keto diet and what it can do to help in the treatment of this disease. A cancer-specific keto diet may consist of as much as 90 percent fat. There is an excellent reason for that. What doctors do know is that cancer cells feed off carbohydrates and sugar. This is what helps them grow and multiply in number.

As we have seen, the keto diet dramatically reduces our carbohydrate and sugar consumption as our metabolism is altered. What the keto diet does, in essence, is to remove the "food" on which cancer cells feed and starves them. The result is that cancer cells may die, multiply at a slower rate, or decrease.

Another reason why a keto diet can slow down the growth of cancer cells is that by reducing calories, cancer cells have less energy to develop and grow in the first place. Insulin also helps cells grow. Since the keto diet lowers insulin level, it slows down the growth of tumorous cells.

When on the keto diet, the body produces ketones. While ketones fuel the body, cancerous cells are not. Therefore, a state of ketosis may help reduce the size and growth of cancer cells.

One study monitored the growth of tumors in patients who have cancer of the digestive tract. Of those patients who received a high carbohydrate diet, tumors showed a 32.2 percent in growth. Patients on a keto diet showed a 24.3 percent growth in their tumor. The difference is quite significant.

Another study involved five patients who combined chemotherapy with a keto diet. Three of these patients went into remission. Two patients saw a progression of the disease when they went off the keto diet.

More studies are needed, but these numbers are encouraging. The keto diet may help prevent cancer from occurring in diabetic patients in the first place. People with diabetes have a higher risk level to develop cancer due to elevated blood sugar levels. Since the ketogenic diet is extremely effective at decreasing the levels of blood sugar, it may prevent the initial onset of cancer.

From what research has discovered so far, the ketogenic diet may:

1. Stop the growth of cancer cells.
2. Help replace cancerous cells with healthy cells.

3. Change the body's metabolism and enable the body to "starve" cancer cells by depriving them of needed nutrition.
4. By lowering the body's insulin level, the ketogenic body may prevent the onset of cancer cells.

On a ketogenic diet specifically for cancer, your fats should be 75 to 90 percent, protein 15-20 percent, and less than 5 percent carbohydrates.

Foods to Eat

- Egg, including yolks
- All green, leafy vegetables, as well as cauliflower, avocado, mushrooms, peppers, cucumbers, and tomatoes.
- When choosing dairy, opt for a full-fat version of cheeses, butter, sour cream, yogurt, and milk.
- Eat nuts such as walnuts, almonds, filberts, and sunflower and pumpkin seeds.

Foods to Eat in Moderation

- Have one serving of root vegetables, such as yams, parsnip, carrots, and turnips per day.
- Fruits contain sugar, so treat them like candy.
- A glass of dry wine, vodka, whiskey, and brandy once a week. Do not drink cocktails with sugars.
- A small piece of chocolate with 75 percent or higher cocoa content once a week.

Foods to Avoid

- Any food containing sugar, including cereals; soft drinks, juices, and sports drinks, candies, and chocolate. Limit artificial sweeteners as much as possible.
- Also starchy food such as pasta and potatoes, bread, potato chips, and french fries, cooking oils, and margarine.
- All beers.

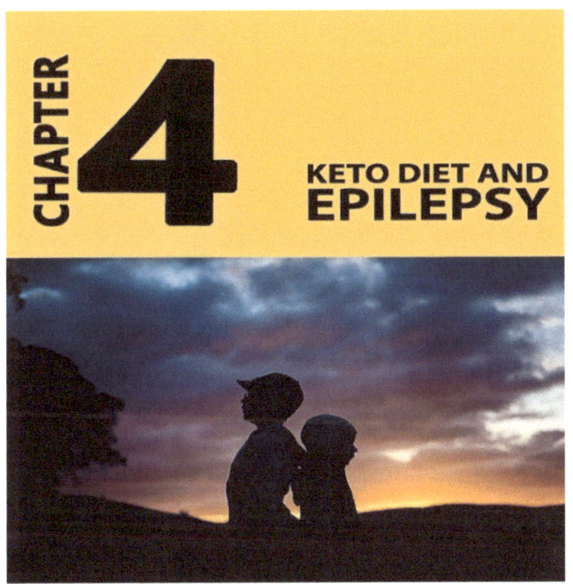

The Keto Diet and Epilepsy

The initial use of the keto diet had nothing to do with weight loss or diabetes management, which it is well known for today. Instead, a doctor created the diet in 1924 to help his patients suffering from epilepsy.

Epilepsy is a nervous system disorder that can bring on recurrent seizures at any time. The symptoms can be spasms and convulsions, or an unusual psychological view of the world. In any case, it is caused by abnormal brain activity. The severity of the symptoms varies from person to person. A person is diagnosed with epilepsy only if he or she suffers from more than two seizures in one full day. Anyone can suffer from this disorder, but it seems to affect young children the most, perhaps because the adolescent brain is still in a state of development.

Drugs frequently manage seizures. Sometimes they work; sometimes, they do not. As far back as 1924, however, Dr. Russell Wilder of the Mayo Clinic conducted groundbreaking research and created the ketogenic diet to help children suffering from epilepsy. It was remarkably effective, but doctors lost interest when new anti-seizure medications came on the market. It was easier for them to prescribe medication than to discuss diet.

However, people who used the keto diet to treat seizures continued seeing remarkable success. Today, doctors are returning to using the low carbohydrate, high-fat diet to treat their patients. The results have been extremely promising.
In 1998, the Journal of Pediatrics published a study involving 150 children who experienced seizures despite taking popular anti-seizure medications. The children were placed on the ketogenic diet

for one year which the researchers assessed their progress.

Eighty-three percent of the subjects were still in the study after three months. Over one-third of the children showed a 90 percent decrease in seizures. At the end of the year, slightly more than half of the subjects had remained on the diet, and a quarter of them experienced a 90 percent decrease in seizures. The numbers indicate that the keto diet has a tremendously positive effect on children who suffer from seizures. The researchers consider it more effective than medication in many cases.

For anyone with children who experience seizures, the inclusion of a keto diet in the child's treatment should be discussed with his or her physician. Another research on the effects of the keto diet on childhood epilepsy involved 145 children. The children were divided into two groups, with one group being treated with medication while the other group was receiving a ketogenic diet. Seventy-four percent of the ketogenic diet group was successful in reducing seizures.

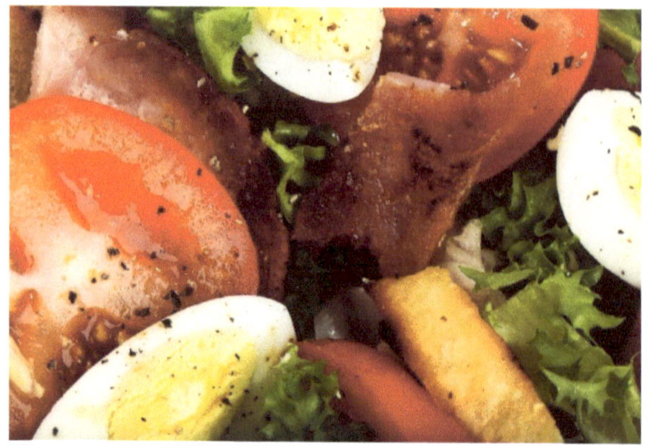

There have been more studies of childhood epilepsy and the keto diet. These have sparked new and considerable interest within the medical profession.

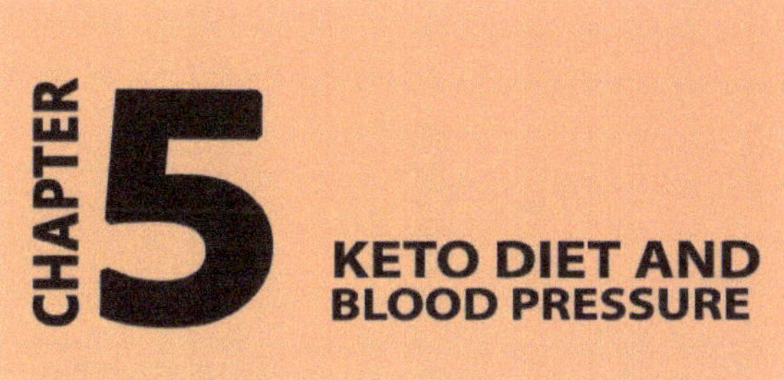

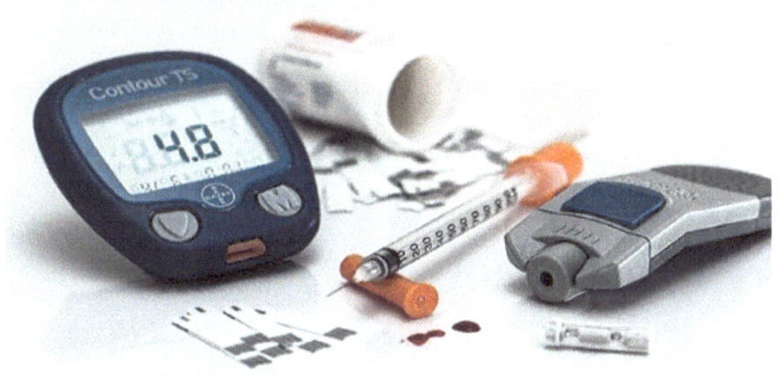

The Keto Diet and Blood Pressure

One-third of American adults suffer from high blood pressure. A severe health problem can lead to heart attacks and strokes. Apparently, the higher the blood pressure, the higher the risk. Aging and obesity significantly increase the chances of developing high blood pressure.

Blood pressure is treated with a variety of medications, some of which can have side effects. The best blood pressure is 120/80. High blood pressure is the result of hypertension, and the causes are not always precise, but we live in an increasingly tense world, and more and more people are dealing with high blood pressure.

It is a known fact that people suffering from high blood pressure frequently carry excess belly fat and can become at risk for type 2 diabetes. To get at the root of all these problems may require a change in lifestyle. An overload of carbohydrates can cause the symptoms of high blood pressure in the diet, more than the body can handle. As we have discussed, carbohydrates are converted into sugars, which raise the body's blood sugar level, forcing the body to create additional insulin. Insulin stores fat, and an excess of insulin can lead to obesity. All of this can have an adverse effect on your blood pressure.

Consuming fewer carbohydrates decreases both the level of insulin and the blood pressure level. This simple dietary change can make a huge difference in your blood pressure.

In a fascinating study released in the Archives of Internal Medicine, 146 overweight people took part in a weight-loss experiment. The people were divided into two groups. One group was put on a ketogenic diet containing a maximum of 20 grams of carbohydrates, while the other group was given the weight-loss drug Orlistat, in addition to being counseled to follow a low-fat regimen.

Both groups showed similar weight loss. What surprised the researchers was that half of the keto group showed a decrease in blood pressure, while only 21 percent of the low-fat diet group had any reduction in blood pressure. While weight loss itself would bring about a lowering of blood pressure, the study suggests that a decrease in carbohydrate intake can help lower blood pressure even more.

It was found that potassium specifically had a significant effect on lower hypertension. Doctors recommend at least 4,700 mg of potassium each day for anyone wishing to lower his or her blood pressure.

Foods high in potassium are:

- Avocado
- Acorn squash
- Bananas
- Coconut water
- Dried apricots

- Pomegranate
- Salmon
- Spinach
- Sweet potato
- White beans

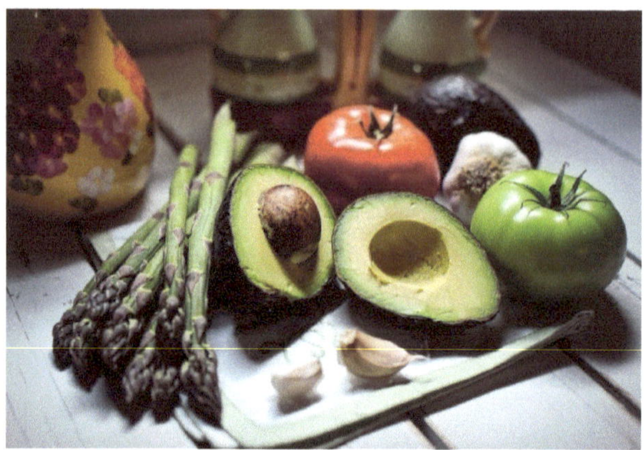

While all these foods are permitted on the ketogenic diet, limit your intake of sweet potato and beans, which are starchy and can contain a high level of carbs.

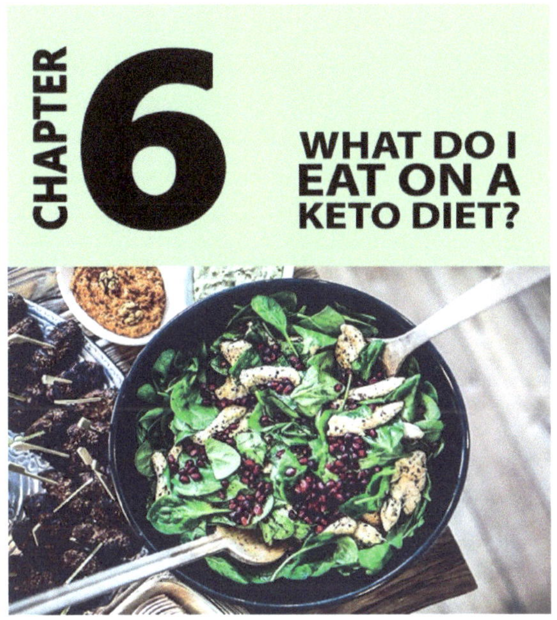

What Do I Eat on The Keto Diet?

Some people associate the keto diet with the bad word "Fat," and are quick to dismiss it. Nothing could be further from the truth. Fat *is* allowed because it is converted into energy. Our body needs healthy fats to thrive. Other foods on the diet could not be healthier. When you are eating ketogenic, you are filling your body with nutrition. Let us look at the foods you will be eating.

As this book has already pointed out, the elimination of processed foods and sugar is one of the best things you can do for your health in general. Processed foods are filled with toxic preservatives that do nothing for you but rob you of your good health. Fresh is always better. When purchasing anything at the market, get into the habit of reading labels. They can be very sneaky and revealing.

Keep your carbohydrates under 50 grams a day, and you will feel the difference. A stricter ketogenic diet will contain approximately 20 grams of carbs a day.

Food to Eat on a Ketogenic Diet

1. Seafood

Everyone knows about the healthy fatty acids, vitamins, and minerals in seafood. Very few of us eat enough. The keto diet encourages the consumption of all things from the sea. Shrimp and crabs are carb-free, and other shellfish contain only a low amount of carbohydrates.

Fatty fish, such as salmon and sardines, are highly recommended because of their high omega-fatty acid content. Fish indeed is brain food. Enjoy at least two servings or more of seafood a week on the keto diet. Simple canned tuna counts as seafood.

2. Vegetables

Can a diet that recommends unlimited green, leafy vegetables be anything but healthy? They are extremely low in carbohydrates and bursting with vitamins, antioxidants, and the fiber we need daily. Green vegetables such as broccoli, spinach, and kale are believed to decrease the risk of heart diseases and cancer. Cauliflower and turnips can be prepared to look and taste like rice or mashed potatoes, with much less starch and carbohydrates.

"Starchy" vegetables, such as potatoes or beets do have carbs and should be limited on the keto diet.

3. Dairy Foods

There are cheeses to satisfy everyone's taste. They are high in fat content for energy, high in protein and calcium, and low in carbohydrates.

Yogurt and cottage cheese are an excellent source of protein and calcium. They are low-carb and fit well into the ketogenic lifestyle. Be sure to stick with plain yogurt, as the flavored types contain much sugar, as are the so-called "low fat" versions of yogurt. You can flavor yogurt and cottage cheese yourself with a few berries and nuts.

4. Avocados

Avocados are true "superfood." They are high in essential vitamins and minerals, including potassium. According to a study, avocados are also believed to help lower cholesterol by 22 percent.

It is also loaded with nutrients and delicious taste; avocados only have 2 grams of net carbohydrates. Use them in salads and sandwiches.

5. Meat and Poultry

The keto diet lets you eat plenty of meat. Meat contains very few carbs and is high in protein to help you build muscles. Whenever possible, choose healthy, grass-fed meats, which are higher in fatty acids.

6. Eggs

Eggs are high in protein and contain a mere 1 gram of carbohydrates. As they are also inexpensive, they are ideal for anyone on a ketogenic diet. Eggs also make you feel full, thereby helping you eat less. Many people take pride in only consuming the whites of eggs, but the right nutrition lies in the yolk, so be sure to eat the egg in its entirety.

7. Coconut Oil

Too many people are unfamiliar with coconut oil, another "superfood." It is perfect for people dealing with diabetes and has been used with Alzheimer patients.

Coconut oil can be used in most recipes in place of butter or oil. You can also use it for frying and sauté.

8. Dark Chocolate

Did you know that dark chocolate has a high amount of antioxidants? Dark chocolate is reaching superfood status. Chocolate with 80 percent or higher real cocoa powder can lower your blood pressure. An ounce of 80 percent dark chocolate contains 10 grams of carbohydrates, so it counts as a healthy snack. Keep in mind the lower of cocoa content, the less healthy the chocolate will be. Milk chocolate does not count as healthy chocolate.

Foods to Avoid on a Ketogenic Diet

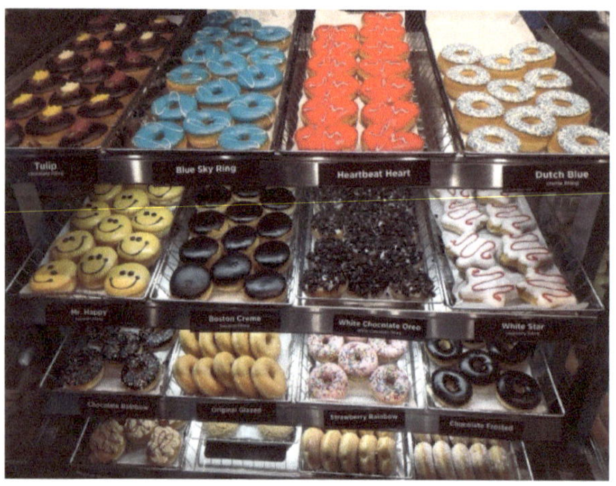

The keto diet has a lot less restricted foods than many other diets. Sugar, of course, should be avoided. That does not mean you cannot enjoy sweet desserts. Many keto-friendly recipes substitute unsweetened applesauce for sugar in baked goods. Substitute sweeteners such as Stevia can use in moderation.

Keep in mind that fruits are healthful, but they do contain a great deal of sugar, so limit the amount you eat to just a few slices a day. Fruit juices are concentrates that have vitamins but lack fiber. Also, their sugar content is extremely high. Read the label on any bottle of juice before buying. The best juices are "green" with just a hint of fruit for flavoring.

Be careful with cereals. Most are packed with sugar and robbed of any nutrients. Many claims, "nutrition added," but all that means is that all nutrition has been removed and replaced with a small amount, and a whole lot of sugar for taste. One hundred percent bran cereal will fit into your keto diet, and you can sweeten it with a handful of berries. Just be sure to examine all labels in the cereal aisle. They can be very tricky. Also, remember that honey, too, is considered as sugar.

Entirely omit white starches from your diet. They are nothing but empty calories. This includes white bread, pasta, and rice. Buy the wholegrain version, instead, and enjoy in moderation.

Legumes and beans are healthy for you, but they are high in carbohydrates. You can have them occasionally; make sure you keep it within your daily 20 – 50 carb-gram count.

Alcohols tend to be empty calories, but certain spirits will be better for you than others will. Beer is filled with carbs and should be off your keto diet. The expression "beer belly" exists for a reason. Enjoy a glass of wine, instead. Of course, there are variances in different types of wine. Dry wines contain a minimum amount of sugar, while sweet dessert wines contain much more.

Pure alcohol such as whiskey and vodka are carb-free, but they do contain calories, so have a care. Mixing alcohol for fancy cocktails usually creates a haven for sugar, so avoid those.

Wine coolers may be a tasty treat, but in reality, they are just sugary sodas with some added alcohol. They should not be on your keto diet at any time.

7

KETO DIET FOR RAPID WEIGHT LOSS

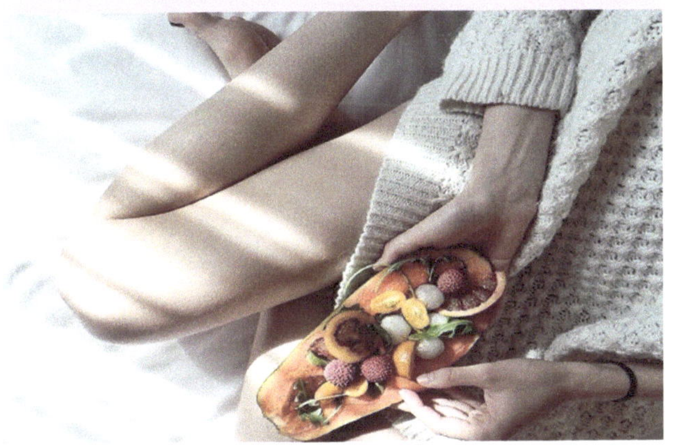

The Keto Diet for Rapid Weight Loss

Many people confuse the ketogenic diet with low carb diets or paleo diets. However, there are considerable differences of which you should be aware.

Keto v. Low Carb

A low-carb diet can be anything it wants to be, as long as it is low in carbohydrates.

Also, "low" is rarely defined. On a low-carb diet, you merely make random food choices that curb your carb intake arbitrarily. Since there is no real number, you might still be consuming too many carbs.

Most importantly, what the low-carb diet lacks is that all-critical ketonic state that turns carbs into fats and provides your body with a new and useful source of fuel. This can leave you very hungry and tired. The ketogenic diet has a specific ratio of carbs to fats to protein. This manipulation is critical, and it is why a low carb diet will not work as well, if at all.

Keto v. Paleo

The Paleo is also a low-carb-type diet. It is base on the assumption that eating the way our cave dwellers ancestors did, i.e., meat and no carbs, sugars, or grains, is the healthiest type of diet.

There are problems with this reasoning. First, our ancestors never experienced the kind of diseases that we face. The ketogenic diet is specifically a "healing" diet that is meant to benefit the body in many ways and help prevent diseases. The paleo diet does not do that.

Also, the paleo diet is base on eating meat instead of manipulating the ratio of fats, carbohydrates, and protein to achieve a ketonic state that uses fat as fuel.

Ketogenic Diet

Ketogenic is low-carb, but it is much more.

There is a reason why the ketogenic diet has become so popular. It helps improve your overall wellbeing in addition to helping you lose weight. You have more energy during the day, and you feel sated and full, thereby reducing the cravings for unhealthy snacks. In essence, you are eating less, but better. That is what makes the keto diet so unique and successful.

The ketogenic diet is not a magic pill made up by some gurus. Countless studies and testimonials can back the effectiveness of this diet. A scientifically proven method balances your body's fat intake to help achieve optimal weight loss.

By using fat instead of sugar as your primary source of energy, the keto diet induces a state of ketosis, which is achieved when your body stops receiving carbohydrates to turn in glucose. The fewer carbs you consume, the more you force your body to burn fat for energy instead of storing it.

This is why it is possible to lose weight so quickly on the keto diet. It counts carbohydrates instead of calories. Using fats as an additional energy source is what ketosis is all about. A natural state helped our hunter-gatherer ancestors survive in the early days.

They feasted on low-carb foods when they could, and fasted when food was scarce. Fat, was stored and converted into energy during the scarce times. The ketogenic state is a natural human state, which makes the ketogenic diet so powerful and successful. In addition to the benefits of the keto diet, most people enjoy the way it makes them feel better.

Weight loss results on the keto diet differ among individuals, depending on their specific body composition. However, weight loss has been the consistent result of people who have been on the keto diet. The keto diet is known as the best weight-loss diet, as well as the healthiest.

A 2017 study divided Crossfit-training subjects into two groups, with both groups following the physical training, but only one group combined the ketogenic diet with the exercise. The results showed that those on the keto diet decreased their fat mass and weight far more than the other group.

The keto diet group showed an average of 3.5-kilo weight loss, 2.6 percent of body fat, and 2.83 kilos in fat mass, while the other group lost no weight, body fat or fat mass. Both groups showed similar athletic performance ability.

A 2012 study divided overweight children and adolescents into two groups; one was put on a keto diet, the other on a low-calorie diet. As in other keto studies, the children on the keto diet decreased their weight, fat mass, and lowered their insulin levels considerably more than the low-calorie group.

Besides more rapid weight loss, a decided advantage of the keto diet over a low-calorie diet is that people stick to the keto diet. A low-calorie diet will help you lose weight, but you may continuously be feeling hungry and deprived. That is the main reason most diets fail. Hunger and deprivation are not a part of the ketogenic lifestyle.

Ketosis Explained

As we have stated earlier, the keto diet is not magic. It is proven science. Ketosis is a natural occurrence that happens when you do not feed your body enough carbohydrates, and it is forced to look for energy elsewhere.

You have undoubtedly experienced ketosis when you have missed a meal or have exhausted your body with rigorous exercise. Whenever these things happen, your body helps you out by raising its level of ketones. However, most people eat enough sugar and carbs to keep ketosis from happening.

We love our sugar and carbs, no matter how bad they are for us, and our bodies will happily use them as fuel. Also, since our bodies want to help us out, it turns any excess glucose into fat and stores it for future use. Stored fat translated into that ridiculous belly fat that you never want.

The more you restrict your carbohydrate consumption, the more your body will produce ketones. It has no other options. When we limit the number of carbohydrates that we eat, our body will still provide us with energy, but it must turn to another source. Also, that alternate source is fat that was stored for emergencies. The result is a state of ketosis. It happens when our body breaks down the fat into fatty acids and glycerol.

Researchers have discovered most of what they know about ketosis from people who fast, thereby depriving them of all sources of energy. After two days of fasting, the body is starting to produce ketones as it breaks down the available protein and begins to use stored fat for fuel. Ketosis is the natural process the body goes through when deprived of other sources of energy.

Going on a ketogenic, diet is healthier than fasting. Ketogenic should become a lifestyle, not a quick weight-loss method. One of the reasons it is so beneficial is that ketones offer protection against diseases and damages that can affect the body. As mentioned before, the keto diet is an excellent tool to prevent many diseases and maintain health and strength longer.

Planning your keto meals will depend largely on your goals. Are you trying to lose weight, or are you on the keto diet to alleviate the symptoms of some disease? The average keto diet will consist of four meals per day, with a total of 100 grams of protein, 25-50 grams of carbohydrates, and 140-160 grams of fat. This can, of course, be adjusted to your personal needs.

For example, if you are on a keto diet to improve cognitive functions, you may want to raise your fat intake to 90 grams a day for optimal results.

Benefits of Intermittent Fasting on Keto

The science behind the ketogenic diet is that the body burns fat when deprived of other sources of fuel. Intermittent fasting is a deliberate deprivation of food and takes the concept a step further. We are not talking long-term fasting.

Intermittent fasting while on a keto diet meant having two meals a day or fasting for one day a week. The fasting time gives the body a chance to rest and rid itself of toxins. It provides an extra boost to the weight-loss benefits of keto and is a great way to jump-start the diet. For weight loss, the keto diet, combined with intermittent fasting, will help you reach your goal faster and easier.

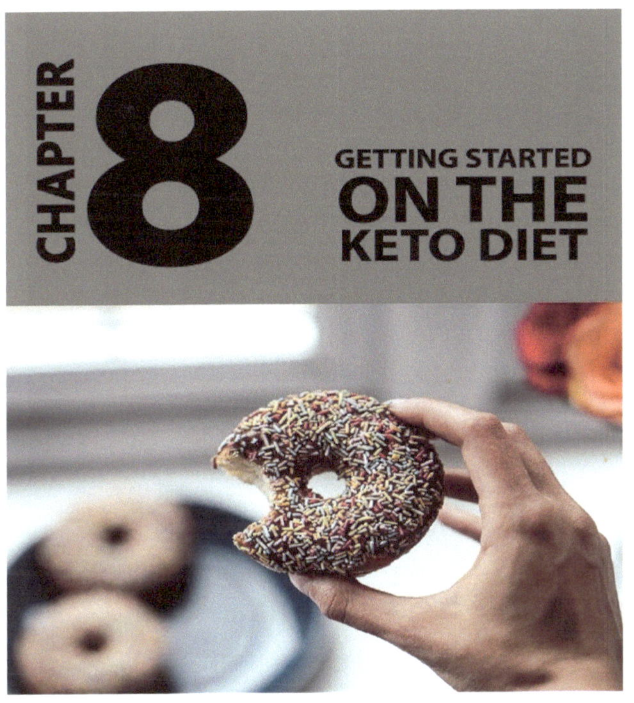

Getting Started on the Keto Diet

Congratulation! You are ready for a new and improved you. There are many excellent benefits to the ketogenic diet. You can expect many positive changes, both physical and mental. So, let us not delay and get the journey started.

Clear Your Pantry

We are sure you have plenty of willpower, but there is no need to confront a kitchen filled with tempting sugars and carbohydrates. Make a clean sweep and pack the offending items in a box. Then donate the loot to a needy neighbor or a soup kitchen. They will appreciate your gesture, and you are on your way to a keto lifestyle. If you have a family, try to get them involved. If they refuse to refrain from eating carbs and sugar, at least insist they do so away from home. It is a fair request.

Weigh Yourself

The keto diet does not require you to live by the tyranny of the scale. As you build up healthy muscles, you might notice a slight initial gain. That is great, so do not worry. You should also have an idea of what your starting point is. If you opted for the keto diet solely to lose weight, you would be able to track your progress. However, do not become a slave to the scale. The occasional weigh-in, perhaps once a week, is enough.

What about Your Favorite Meals?

Perhaps the very thought of giving up your favorite foods has prevented you from getting started on the keto way of life. Relax. The truth is, for every dish that you love and cannot live without (yes that includes cheesecake and mashed potatoes!), you can easily find a low-carb substitute that is just as tasty.

First, let us consider items at your market labeled "low carbohydrate." Labels are frustratingly deceiving, and you would have to be a nutritional expert to understand them. All-too-frequently, off-the-shelf low carb products have simply substituted sugar for carbs, so do not fall for that bit of deceit. You need to learn to read labels with the diligence that you would read your wealthy uncle's will, but your best bet is to stay away from these products and find healthier substitutes. The same goes for anything labeled "low fat," which inevitably means added sugars.

If you are craving a taco? Use a lettuce wrap instead of a taco shell. Do you want rice or mashed potatoes? Grate or rice a cauliflower, and you will not be able to tell the difference. Can't give up your favorite pasta dish? Turn zucchini into "zoodles" by slicing it or using a spiral cutter and enjoy your pasta. If you have to have your favorite dessert on the keto diet, you can. Just bake with almond flour and use unsweetened applesauce and avocado to create some sweet smoothness.

Learn about coconut oil, which you can use as a butter substitute in sautéing, frying, and baking. Coconut oil has incredible health benefits, especially for Type-2 diabetics.

On the keto diet, you will be able to enjoy all your favorite meals, only better.

Always Stay Hydrated

The keto diet tends to lower your insulin level, so your kidneys may be excreting more liquid than usual. Be sure to drink plenty of water.

Condiments Can Be the Enemy

Do not assume condiments do not count on a diet. On the keto diet, they most certainly do. Ketchup has a lot of sugar. Not all salad dressings are equal. Read the label, and never opt for the "fat-free" version. They have merely substituted sugar for fat.

Ordering salads when eating out is one of your best options but beware of the dressing that the restaurant serves. Either ask about the ingredients or better, bring your salad dressing. Do not hesitate to do that, even in a posh eatery where the Maître d' might become spastic at the sight of you pulling salad dressing out of your bag.

Keep Track of Your Ketone Level

It is especially important to remain aware of how your body is responding to the keto diet at the start of the diet. You can do so by doing a simple urine test. You can also purchase a blood ketone meter. It is recommended to perform the test early in the morning.

Friends and Family can be Annoying Bless Their Hearts

Those nearest and dearest to you may not always understand what you are doing. When eating as a group, they may put subtle pressure on you to "just try a bite," or "one slice of cake won't kill you." Or worse, "but I cooked it especially for you!"

It will take resolve to stick to your diet. It may help to fill up on keto-friendly snacks before you sit down and eat. Enjoy some nuts, an avocado, or just a leg of chicken *before* you eat, and you will be less tempted.

Celebrate!

Celebratory occasions, especially if you are the guest of honor, can be a huge hurdle. When the gang at the office or your parents enter a room with a cake yelling "Surprise!" on your birthday, it is hard to refuse. So, try being a bit sneaky, instead.

By all means, gush over the offering. You are expected to do that. You can even help cut slices. Then, discover a sudden and irresistible urge for coffee, which you verbalize loudly and clearly. Gently remove yourself from the center of activity to get coffee for yourself and anyone else. By the time, anyone notices, hopefully, they have missed the fact that you have not eaten anything.

Traveling

Traveling while on the keto diet can be a challenge, so be prepared. Pack a personal blender with some avocados and bananas for a few quick and healthful smoothies. Pack some anchovies or tuna for protein.

Eating Out

Eating out is not as difficult as you may think. Even fast-food places have salads, these days. In any restaurant, stick to meat and vegetables and forego the potatoes and noodles.

You can even navigate the tricky maze in a Chinese restaurant. While abstaining from rice, you can enjoy the following: clear soups, steamed fish with vegetables, egg foo young, stir-fried dishes, Mu Shu without the wrappers are just a few suggestions. Ask your server if your meal can be prepared without cornstarch, which is used as a thickener.

Even if you end up in a fast food place, that does not have salad, toss the buns from your burger and eat the meat. You can do the same at a friend's house or a BBQ.

Exercise

The keto diet will build muscle mass and give you added energy. Do not forget to incorporate exercise into your daily routine. It can be as simple as walking more, taking the stairs, or joining a gym.

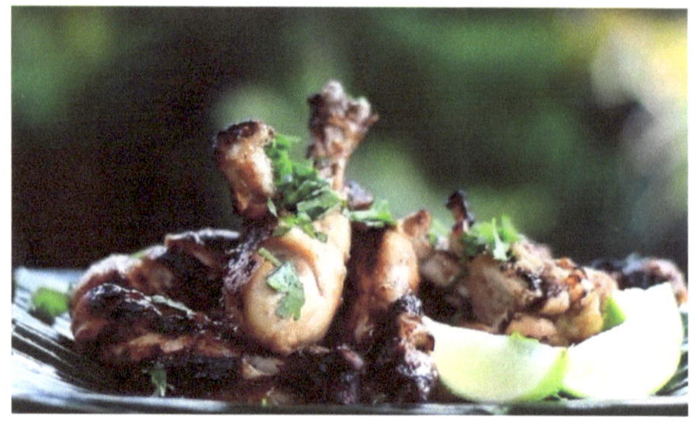

How Long Should You Stay on a Ketogenic Diet"

The amount of time spent on the diet can vary and should be discussed with your doctor. Many people who use the ketogenic diet for weight loss remain on the diet for several weeks, until they have achieved a goal, then they turn to a paleo diet or other maintenance eating. You do not want to lose weight only to return to your old eating habits.

If you are on the ketogenic diet for medical or therapeutic reasons, check with your doctor to ascertain if you should remain on the diet for a more extended period.

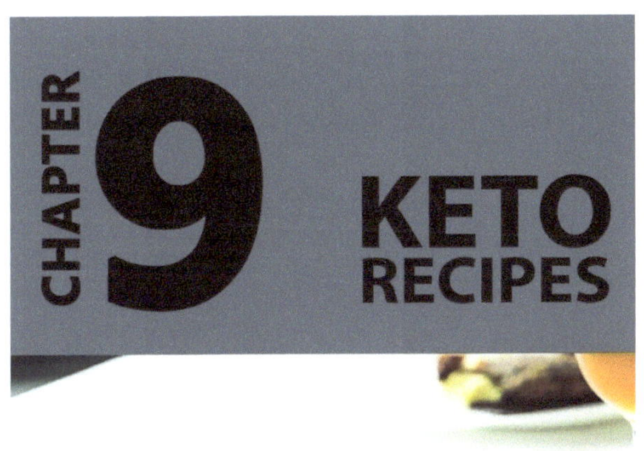

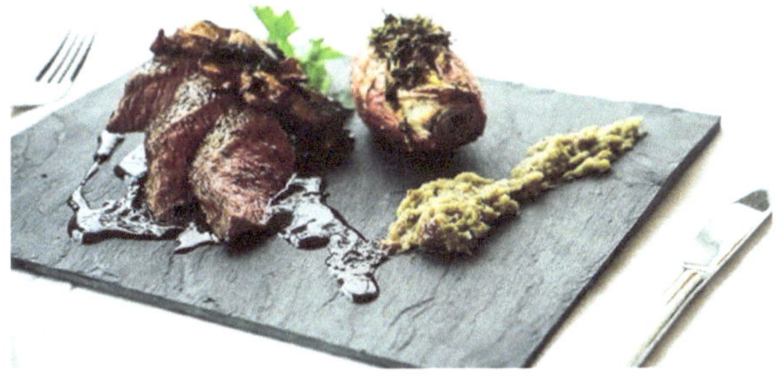

Keto Recipes

You can take your favorite recipes and turned them "keto." Below are a few recipes to show you how easy it is. It might be an excellent idea to buy a keto cookbook for your kitchen.

Two of the essential keto recipes are the simple cauliflower rice and "zoodles." They could not be easier to prepare. People can get frustrated with the keto diet when they crave pasta and rice. These two recipes definitely satisfy those cravings; they taste just like the real thing. The zoodles can be used for any pasta dish.

Omelet Muffins

Make plenty of these ahead of time. They will go fast.

Ingredients:
- 1 tbsp. butter
- 10 eggs
- Salt and pepper to taste
- ½ cup diced ham
- ¼ cup drained spinach
- ¼ cup diced onion
- ¼ cup chopped red bell pepper
- ¼ cup shredded Pepper Jack cheese

Directions:
1. Preheat the oven to 350 degrees.
2. Coat a muffin pan with non-stick spray.
3. Whisk the eggs, and then stir in the remaining ingredients.
4. Fill the muffin pan with the mixture
5. Bake for 25 minutes.
6. Nutritional Facts: Calories 155; carb. 2 g; fat 10 g; protein 12.5 g.

Breakfast Casserole

This is a delicious casserole everyone can enjoy. It will leave you satisfied until lunch.

Ingredients:
- 10 eggs
- ¼ cup whipping cream
- 1 cup ricotta cheese
- 1 diced onion
- Salt and pepper to taste
- 1 package thawed frozen spinach
- 1 cup sliced mushrooms
- 1 lb. crumbled sausage meat

Directions:
1. Preheat oven to 350 degrees.
2. Whisk the eggs, whipping cream, ricotta cheese, and onion well
3. Season with salt and pepper.
4. Add the spinach, mushrooms, and crumbled sausage.
5. Bake for 30 minutes.

Keto Pancakes

Serve these pancakes with butter and sugar-free syrup or with berries.

Ingredients:
- 1 ¼ cup almond flour
- 2 tbsp. honey

- Dash of salt
- 1 tsp. baking powder
- 1 tsp. cinnamon
- 6 beaten eggs
- ¼ cup plain Greek yogurt
- 3 tbsp. melted butter
- 1 tsp. lemon extract

Directions:
1. Stir the flour, baking powder, and cinnamon in a bowl.
2. Combine the eggs, honey, yogurt, lemon extract and butter in another bowl.
3. Slowly stir the egg mixture into the flour mixture.
4. Use two tablespoons of batter and drop on a hot griddle.
5. Cook for 4 minutes, then flip and cook for another 2 minutes.
6. Continue until all batter has been used.
7. Nutritional Information: 413 calories; 34 g fat; 18.4 g carbohydrates; 16.3 g protein.

Apple Red Cabbage

Cabbage is a great vegetable to have on keto. This red cabbage side dish is yummy.

Ingredients:
- 8 slices of bacon, cut into pieces

- 1 large diced onion
- 1 peeled and sliced the apple
- 2 cup chicken broth
- 3 tbsp. red cider vinegar
- 2 tbsp. coconut palm sugar or sugar substitute, such as Splenda
- 1 tsp. ground cloves
- ½ tsp. allspice
- ½ tsp. nutmeg
- Salt and pepper to taste
- 1 shredded red cabbage

Directions:
1. Fry the bacon in a skillet until crispy.
2. Add the onion and sauté for 5-6 minutes.
3. Stir in the broth, sugar, vinegar, spices, salt, and pepper.
4. Add the cabbage and cook on low for 45 minutes.
5. Nutrition Facts: 160 calories; 7.8 g fat; 16 g carbohydrates; 4 g protein.

Cinnamon Granola

Store-bought granola usually has high sugar content. Try this instead.

Ingredients:
- 1 cup chopped walnuts

- ½ cup shredded coconuts
- ¼ cup sliced almonds
- 2 tbsp. Sunflower seeds
- ½ tsp. cinnamon
- 1 tbsp. coconut palm sugar
- 1 tbsp. melted butter

Directions:
1. Preheat the oven to 375 degrees.
2. Combine the walnuts, shredded coconut, sliced almonds, and sunflower seeds.
3. Add cinnamon and coconut palm sugar and stir into the nut mixture.
4. Spread the mixture in a single layer on a baking sheet.
5. Drizzle with the melted butter.
6. Bake for 20 minutes.
7. Nutrition Facts: 180 calories; 19 g fat; 4.1 g carbohydrates; 4 g protein.

Herbed Omelet with Smoked Salmon

You can enjoy this omelet anytime, but a breakfast of protein and fatty acids gets the day started right.

Ingredients:
- 2 tbsp. butter
- 2 beaten eggs
- 1 tsp. tarragon

- 1 tsp. thyme
- Salt and pepper to taste
- 1 tbsp. butter
- 2 tbsp. chopped onions
- 4 very thin tomato slices
- 2 smoked salmon sliced
- 1 tsp. capers

Directions:
1. Whisk the eggs and add the tarragon, thyme, salt, and pepper.
2. Melt the butter in a skillet and add the beaten eggs and chopped onions.
3. Cook for 3-4 minutes, until the eggs begin to set.
4. Transfer the omelet to a plate and top with the tomato and salmon slices. Sprinkle with capers.
5. Nutrition Facts: Calories: 239; fat 15 g; carbohydrates 4 g; protein 22 g.

Cheeseburger Salad

This is your favorite cheeseburger without the bun.

Ingredients:
- 1 lb. ground beef
- Salt and pepper to taste
- 3 cups chopped lettuce
- 1 small diced onion

- 1 sliced tomato
- ¼ cup shredded cheddar cheese
- 4 tbsp. oil and vinegar dressing

Directions:
1. Fry the ground beef in a skillet for 4 minutes.
2. Add the onion and cook for another 5 minutes.
3. Place the beef and onions in a bowl and add the remaining ingredients, except the dressing.
4. Coat with the salad dressing.
5. Nutrition Facts: Calories 290; Fat 14 g; Carbohydrates 6; Protein 25 g.

Cauliflower Rice

This straightforward recipe is for basic rice. You can dress it up with vegetables, spices, or stir-fry it. Use this anytime you need rice as a side dish or in a recipe.

Ingredients:
- 1 cauliflower head

Directions:
1. Chop the cauliflower into florets.
2. Place the florets in a food processor and pulse until you have a rice-like consistency.
3. Cook the rice in a pan of salted water for 5 minutes.

4. Nutritional Facts: Calories 21; Carbohydrates 5; Fat 0; Protein 0

Zoodles

These zoodles made from zucchini taste like noodles. A spiralizer is the easiest way to create zoodles, but you can also use a mandolin. Zoodles get soggy very quickly, so do not cook for more than 1 minute. Season with butter or shredded cheese.

Ingredients:
- 1 zucchini

Directions:
1. Use a spiralizer to create pasta strands.
2. Bring a pot of salted water to boil and cook the zoodles for 1 minute.

Bacon-Wrapped Chicken

A very decadent and delicious way to enjoy chicken.

Ingredients:
- 2 lbs. boneless and skinless chicken breast
- 2 cups chopped spinach
- 1 cup sliced mushrooms
- 1 cup cream cheese
- ½ cup cottage cheese

- Salt and pepper to taste
- 12 slices bacon

Directions:
1. Preheat the oven to 375 degrees
2. Combine the spinach, mushroom, cream cheese and cottage cheese in a bowl.
3. Season the mixture with salt and pepper.
4. Use a mallet to flatten the chicken pieces to a 1/2 -inch thickness.
5. Use a sharp knife to cut pockets in one end.
6. Spoon the mixture into the pockets.
7. Wrap two bacon slices around each chicken piece.
8. Brown the wrapped chicken in a skillet 5 minutes each side.
9. Place the chicken pieces in a baking dish.
10. Bake the chicken for 45 minutes. The bacon should be crispy, and the chicken is done.
11. Nutrition Facts: Calories 390; Fat 22 g; Carbs 3.9 g; Protein 41 g.

Cobb Salad

This salad is very high in protein. Enjoy.

Ingredients for Dressing:
- 1 tbsp. olive oil

* 1 tbsp. white vinegar
* 1 tsp. Dijon mustard
* 2 tbsp. diced onion
* Salt and pepper to taste

Ingredients for Cobb Salad:
* ¾ cup cubed cooked chicken
* ½ cup diced tomatoes
* ½ cup blue cheese
* 2 tablespoons blue cheese
* 1 sliced hard-boiled egg
* 2 cups chopped greens
* 1 sliced avocado
* 4 cooked and sliced bacon slices

Directions:
1. Arrange the greens on a plate
2. Arrange rows of chicken, diced tomatoes, blue cheese, egg slices, avocado slices and bacon pieces on top of the greens.
3. Combine all the dressing ingredients.
4. Drizzle the dressing over the salad.
5. Nutrition facts: Calories 295; Fat 11 g; Carbs 4 g; Protein 22 g.

Slow Cooker Pot Roast

This pot roast is prepared without potatoes or carrots. If you add them, adjust the carbs accordingly.

Ingredients:

- 2 lb. chuck roast
- Salt and pepper to taste
- 1 tbsp. olive oil
- 2 minced garlic cloves
- 1 chopped onion
- 2 ½ cup beef broth
- ½ cup dry red wine

Directions:

1. Season the roast with salt and pepper.
2. Salt and pepper the roast.
3. Heat the olive oil in a skillet and brown the roast on all sides.
4. Place the roast and remaining ingredients in the slow cooker.
5. Stir the ingredients to combine.
6. Cook on low for 6 hours.
7. Nutrition facts: Calories 242; Fat 12 g; Carbs 9.8 g; Protein 21g.

Spinach and Sausage Soup

This soup is loaded with flavor while remaining very low in carbs.

Ingredients:

- 1 lb. spicy crumbled Italian sausage
- 1 tbsp. olive oil
- 1 chopped onion
- 2 sliced carrots

- 1 minced garlic clove
- 2 tbsp. red wine vinegar
- ½ tsp. oregano
- Dash of hot sauce
- 4 cups chicken broth
- ½ cup whipping cream
- 2 cups baby spinach
- Salt and pepper to taste

Directions:
1. Heat the olive oil in a skillet and saute the crumbled sausage for 5 minutes, until it is no longer pink.
2. Transfer the sausage to a plate and drain on a paper towel.
3. Sauté the onion, garlic, and carrot in the same pan.
4. Deglaze the pan with the red wine vinegar.
5. Add the chicken stock, whipping cream, oregano, and hot sauce and stir well. Season with salt and pepper.
6. Simmer the soup for 5 minutes.
7. Transfer the sausage back into the pan and stir in the spinach.
8. Cook for 1 minute to allow the spinach to wilt.
9. Nutrition facts: Calories 137; Fat 7.8 g; Carbs 2 g; Protein 11g.

Tandoori Chicken

Tandoori chicken is all about the spice marinade. Serve it with some cauliflower rice.

Ingredients:
- 2 lbs. chicken thighs

Ingredients for Marinade:
- 1 cup plain yogurt
- 2 tsp. lemon juice
- Salt and pepper to taste
- 2 tbsp. olive oil
- 2 minced garlic cloves
- 1 tsp. chili powder
- 1 tsp. grated fresh ginger
- 1 tsp. garam masala
- ½ tsp. cumin

Directions:
1. With a sharp knife, cut several slits into the chicken thighs.
2. Season the chicken with salt and pepper and drizzle with the lemon juice.
3. Combine the remaining ingredients in a large bowl.
4. Place the chicken in the bowl and coat thoroughly.
5. Refrigerate up to 24 hours. The longer you marinate, the more flavor is absorbed.

6. Preheat the oven to 375 degrees.
7. Line a baking sheet with aluminum foil and layer the chicken on top.
8. Bake for about 45 – 50 minutes, until the skin is nice and crispy.
9. Nutrition facts: Calories 145; Fat 5.8 g; Carbs 2.3 g; Protein 17g.

Curried Lamb

Filled with exotic spices, this curry dish is perfect with keto rice.

Ingredients:
- 2 lbs. lamb meat
- 1 tbsp. olive oil
- 1 diced onion
- 3 minced garlic cloves
- ½ tsp. grated ginger
- ½ to. turmeric
- ½ tsp. curry powder
- ½ tsp. garam masala
- 2 cups beef stock
- 1 cup plain Greek yogurt
- 1 tsp. lemon juice

Directions:
1. Cut the lamb meat into small pieces
2. Sauté the onion in the olive oil for 5 minutes, then add the garlic, ginger, turmeric, curry powder and garam masala. Stir for another 5 minutes.

3. Add the meat and brown it for 10 minutes.
4. Pour in the beef stock and simmer for 40 minutes.
5. Remove from heat and stir in the yogurt and lemon juice.
6. Nutrition Facts: Calories 329; Fat 17 g; Carbs 9.1 g; Protein 36 g.

Cheddar Biscuits

These tasty biscuits are great anytime. They freeze well, so keep them handy.

Ingredients:
- 2 cups almond flour
- 1 cup shredded cheddar cheese
- 1 cup coconut oil
- 1 cup cream cheese
- 3 eggs
- 2 tsp. baking powder
- 1 tsp. baking soda
- Dash of salt

Directions:
1. Preheat oven to 325 degrees.
2. Cover a baking sheet with aluminum foil.
3. Place the flour and the cheese in a food processor and pulse to a grainy consistency.

4. Add the baking powder and baking soda.
5. Heat the cream cheese and coconut oil in a small pan and warm until they melt. Stir to a creamy smoothness.
6. Whisk the eggs and add the salt.
7. Stir the flour mixture into the egg mixture and stir until a dough forms.
8. Use a tablespoon to drop the dough onto the baking sheet.
9. Bake for 25 minutes.
10. Allow the biscuits to cool for slicing.
11. Nutrition Facts: Calories 106; Fat 11.1 g; Carbs 2 g; Protein 3.9 g.

Conclusion

Congratulations. You have mastered the ketogenic diet. You have lost weight, feel better, look fabulous, and are enjoying an abundance of energy. You have put much effort into improving your health, so what happens when you have reached your goal, and it is time to abandon the keto diet?

It is a fact that maintaining your weight loss can be more difficult than losing that weight in the first place. Returning to your old, bad eating habits may be all-too-tempting. Also, when you discontinue the keto diet, your metabolism is likely to slow down, making weight maintenance more difficult.

You certainly do not want to lose momentum and return to the unhealthy, all-American, sugar and carbohydrate swamp, with your lost weight returning. The options below are undoubtedly best at maintaining your current state of health.

Consider your options before you stop the keto diet. Have a plan in place and execute it. Since the keto diet provides you with many options, it will be easier to adjust to a maintenance style.

Continue Keto

Continue on the keto diet that has been successful for you, but consume more food. Not different, high-carb foods, but the same foods you ate on the diet, in somewhat more substantial quantities. You will be eating more calories.

This will allow you to eat more protein and fats but keep the carbohydrate level low. This can be a hit and miss process; add more calories to your diet and see how your body reacts and adjust accordingly.

This option ensures that carbohydrates are no longer running your life, as you will not suffer from the cravings you might have had when you started the keto diet.

The shift from Losing Weight to Gaining Muscles

With the increasing energy you enjoy on the keto diet, you may wish to focus on improving your muscle tone. Many athletes are fans of the keto diet. This means retaining your low body fat but adding muscle and definition. Strong muscles help strengthen bone density and keep you strong as you age.

The best way to gain strong muscles is to consume more calories in the form of lean proteins. This option is difficult to maintain unless to include a resistance training exercise program.

Remain on Low Carb but not on Keto

When you use the keto diet to lose weight, your carbohydrate restrictions are relatively strict. You can still maintain your weight with a low carb diet, but not as rigid as keto. There are many healthy beans and legumes you can enjoy by adding a few more carbs to your diet.

How much more carbs is very individual because everybody is different. Add a few cups of beans, lentils, or another serving of carrots to your diet each week and see how your body reacts. If you continue to maintain your goal weight, you are on the right track. Add 10 grams of carbohydrates a week until you are satisfied with the results.

The advantage of this option is that it allows you to eat right, healthy foods that were off-limits on the keto diet. Having a greater variety of foods from which to choose will make it easier to maintain your weight.

If you find yourself gaining weight, just cut down on the added carbs just a bit.

Use Intermittent Fasting

Intermittent fasting gives you additional options. Remember that fasting forces your body to burn fat.

Here are some ways you can fast intermittently:

1. Eat what you want for five days, and then fast for two days.
2. Eat two meals a day instead of three, providing for a more extended period where you are not consuming food.

When you begin to embrace keto, you will be enjoying all the benefits of healthy eating. By continuing to consume fewer carbohydrates as a lifestyle, your body will remain sleek and robust. You will also be providing it with ammunition to ward off many chronic diseases.

Many thanks for purchasing and reading my book. In the event that you enjoyed the book, please consider leaving a review on Amazon. I would really appreciate it. All the best on your weight loss journey also to a healthier you. God Bless You!

Love
Annett Hill